DIY Repellents:

Make You Own Non-Toxic Insect Repellents and
After Bite Remedies

Table of Contents

Introduction

Mosquitoes are never welcomed. They make fizzing sounds. They bite too and their bites hurt as well. Pain, itching and swelling all are the unpleasant results of these bites but did you know that there are a number of things in your home that you can use to sooth the feeling such as ice cube, honey and milk.

You like growing ornamental plants and herbs in your home garden but did you know that many of them can repel insects by just staying in your garden beds and smiling at you?! Similarly, did you know that sprinkling water solutions of garlic, mint, basil leaves and lavender can make your house a non-favorite place for many kinds of insects and bugs?!

This book is full of such organic and environment friendly recipes and remedies to repel the flying and crawling gifts of summer from your home. Let's read and try some of the magical antidotes this year!

Chapter 1: Essential Ingredients for Homemade Repellents

Summer is a beautiful season in which everything appears to be brighter and clearer. It is the season of freshness. It is an amazing feeling to go on evening walks in summer days. But there a few not much welcomed gifts other than these as well that summer season brings with it.

One of them is the insects. All kind of insects, bugs, crawlers, flies and mosquitoes grow and breed in summer therefore they are going to hang around you very much. Getting rid of them is easier in this technological era but doing that while staying environment friendly is a little trickier. Here, we will discuss some of the essential elements that you must have in your home to make repellents. But first, we will look at the dos and don'ts for the process;

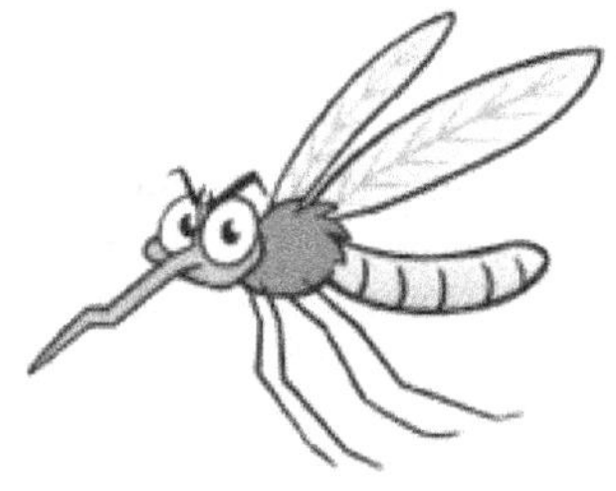

Dos for Repelling Mosquitoes:

1. Hang a mosquito net on your bed before sleeping. Remember that all mosquito repellent lotions and sprays work for a few hours. Their effect decreases afterwards therefore hanging a mosquito net on your bed is a must.

2. Keep all the doors and windows of your house closed especially in summer evenings. It will prevent entry of mosquitoes in your house.

3. Kill all mosquitoes on sight. This will make the environment around relatively mosquito free.

4. Mosquitoes are attracted to light. Therefore use mosquito repellent lights such as LED lights, yellow bug lights and sodium lamps in your house.

Don'ts for Repelling Mosquitoes:

1. Make sure that no water stand inside or near your house. Pungent water is the most favorable place for mosquitoes to lay eggs.

Essential Ingredients for Homemade Repellents:

There is a large variety of all kind of mosquito and bugs repellents available in the market. They are effective but harmful to our environment. Therefore, you must avoid using them. Here are some of the homemade repellents.

1. Herbs:

Herbs provide health benefits in a number of ways. They repel mosquitoes for you as well. Here are some of such herbs for you;

a. Basil:

Basil repels mosquitoes and home flies. You can plant it in containers and place them anywhere indoor or outdoor in your house. Add 4-5 fresh clean basil leaves in 4 ounces of boiling water. Pour it in a spray bottle after removing the leaves. Add 4 ounces of cheap vodka. Spray on your skin avoiding mouth, eyes and nose as a mosquito repellent.

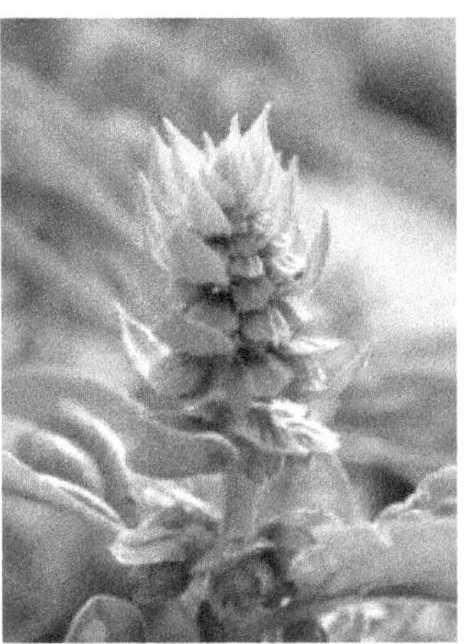

b. Lavender:

It repels mosquitoes, flies, fleas and moths. Simple place its bouquets at different places in your house. You can also use its oil in different ways to make homemade mosquito repellents.

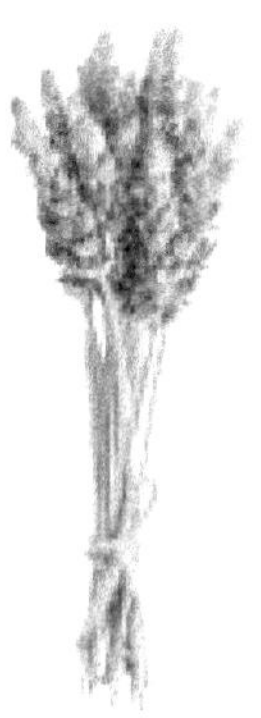

c. Lemongrass:

They greatly repel mosquitoes. Citronella candles are largely found in stores to be burnt for repulsion. It is natural oil found in lemon grass.

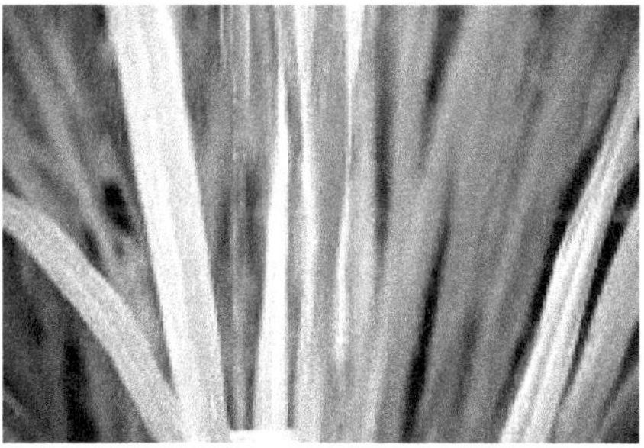

d. Lemon thyme:

This hardy herb repels mosquitoes specifically. It thrives in your garden and can adapt to rocky or dry and shallow soil. Bruise its leaves to release the chemical. Simply take a few leaves and rub them on your hands after crushing them up. Check your tolerance beforehand.

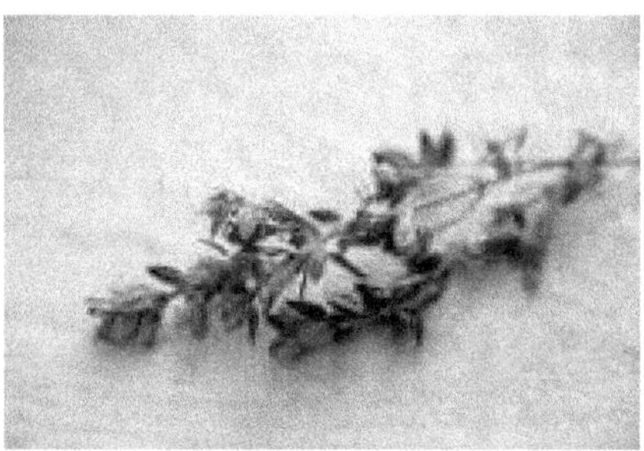

e. Mint:

It greatly repels mosquitoes. It is a perennial herb with a long list of health benefits. To make a mosquito repellent, extract its oil and mix it with cheap vodka and apple cider vinegar. Keep it in a spray bottle. Sprinkle and rub on your body before going into a mosquito prone area.

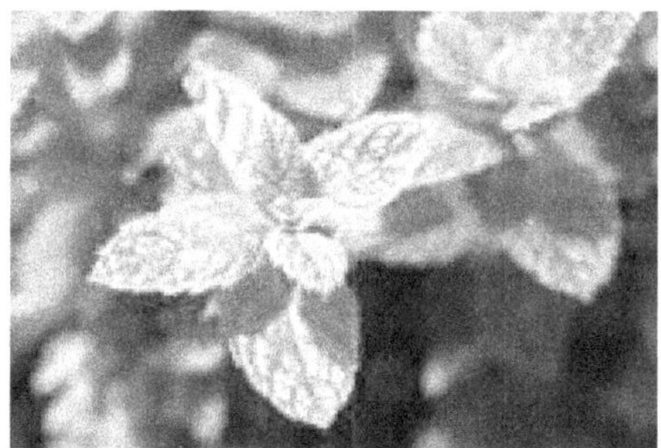

f. Rosemary:

It repels mosquitoes along with a large variety of insects that are harmful to vegetables. Its oil can also be extracted and used in many types of homemade mosquito repellents. Simply boil a portion of dried rosemary in water for 20-30 minutes and put it in refrigerator on cooling down. Take it out and sprinkle the solution in mosquito prone areas of your house.

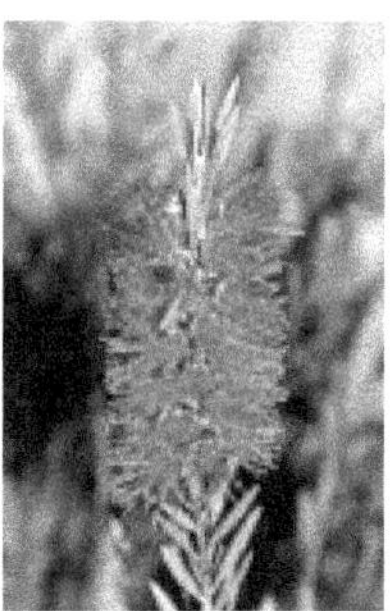

2. Ornamental Flowers:

Ornamental plants really add to the beauty of your home garden. But they are helpful in repelling mosquitoes and other bugs as well. Here are the important ones;

a. Alliums:

They are considered to be broad spectrum insecticides. They repel slugs, cabbage worms, carrot flies, and aphids. They make a great addition in your home garden.

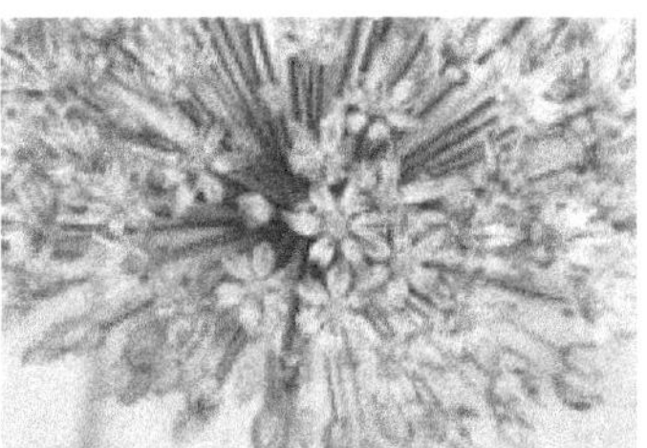

b. Marigolds:

They are great in repelling rabbits, mosquitoes and aphids. Their roots repel nematodes. They make a beautiful addition in your home garden as well.

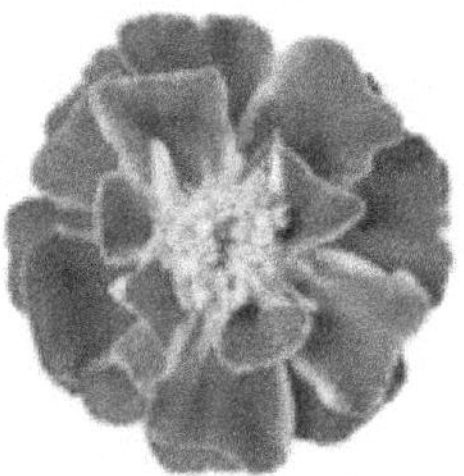

c. Nasturtiums:

They are famous for repelling cabbage loopers, many beetles, aphids, squash bugs and whiteflies. They release an airborne chemical to repel predacious insects. They look beautiful too.

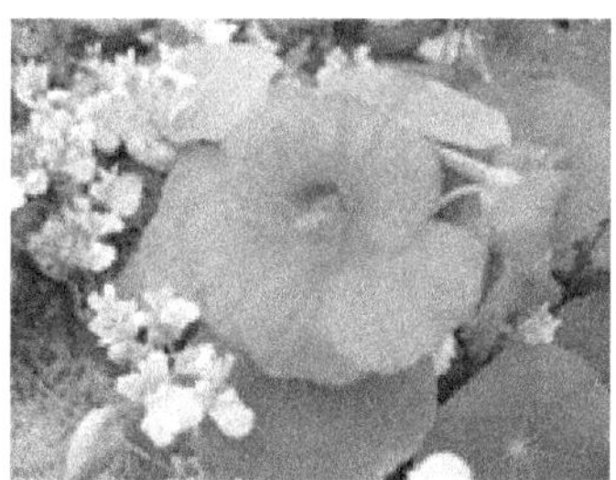

d. Petunias:

They successfully repel squash bugs, leafhoppers, asparagus beetles, tomato hornworms, and aphids. They are popular because of their bright colors as well. They also require minimal maintenance.

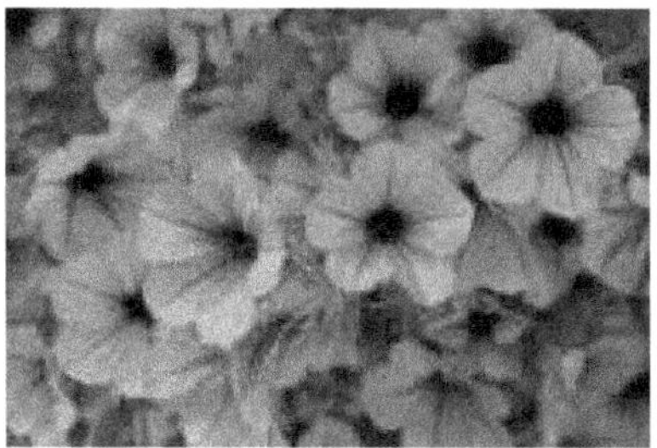

3. Carnivorous Plants:

Mother Nature specifically nurtures some plants to feed on insects and bugs. Some of them are;

a. Pitcher Plants:

They trap and ingest bugs and insects. Their attractive colors and shapes attract insects and the plants trap them in their pitcher which actually is a specialized leaf.

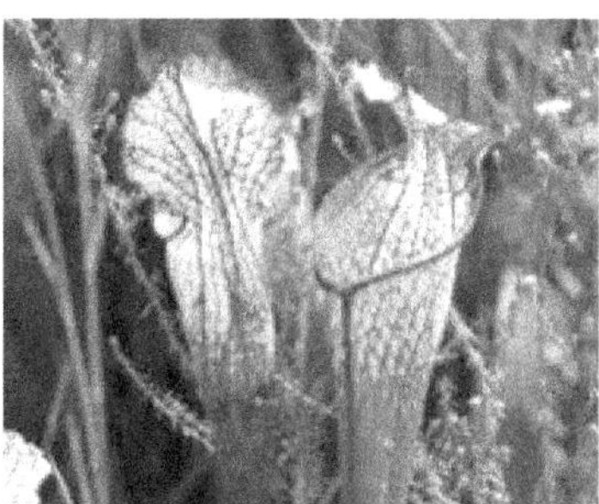

b. Venus Flytrap:

They work on the same principle as the pitcher plants. However, they feed on ants and other insects.

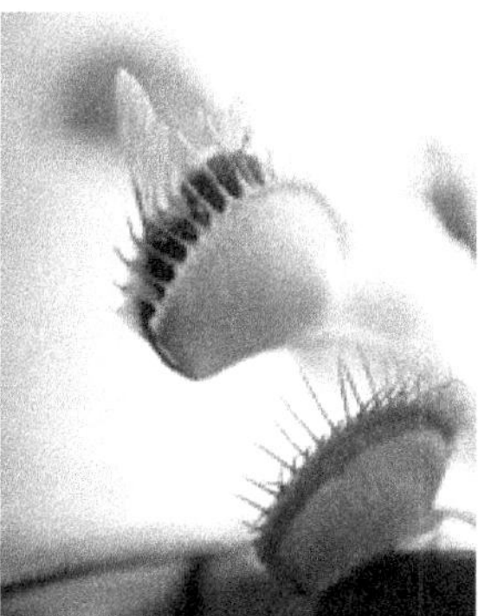

You can grow all or many of these herbs, ornamental plants and carnivorous in your home garden and enjoy an insect free environment friendly ambiance of the indoors.

Chapter 2: Natural Insect Repellents for People

Mosquitoes' job is to suck, literally. And many of your people are mosquito magneto and have to wear an itchy, bumpy skin all the time. There are many reasons that attract mosquitoes to come and bite you such as your body scent, heat, light and humidity. However, different species of mosquitoes get attracted to different aspects such as the ones who carry malaria get attracted to the bacteria and sweat on your skin. Some of them are attracted to certain hand odors and carbon dioxide as well.

Whatever specie is attracted to you, you can use DEET based repellent to protect your skin from the encounter. Most of the government agencies also recommend DEET based repellents as well but these chemical products cause a number of environmental and health problems. Therefore, you must avoid using such kind of harmful products.

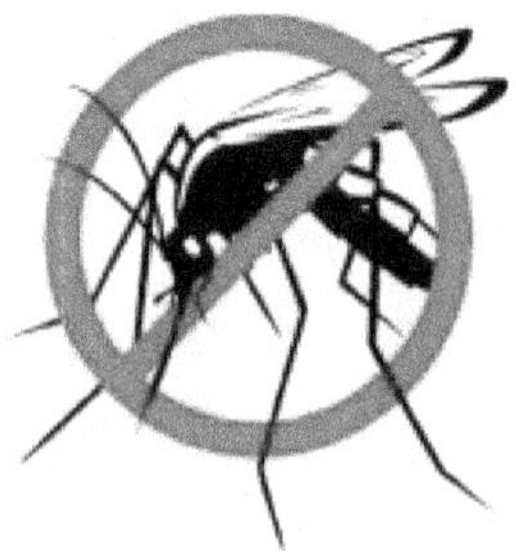

For keeping mosquitoes away from your skin without relying on the harmful products, here we are discussing some natural remedies for this purpose;

1. **Lemon Eucalyptus Oil:**

Lemon eucalyptus oil is a naturally found mosquito repellent. It has been used since 1940s. The Centers of Disease Control and Prevention has also approved it as the most effective among all natural mosquito repellents. A recent scientific study has also proven that only 32% lemon eucalyptus provides more than 95% prevention of mosquito bites for upto three hours.

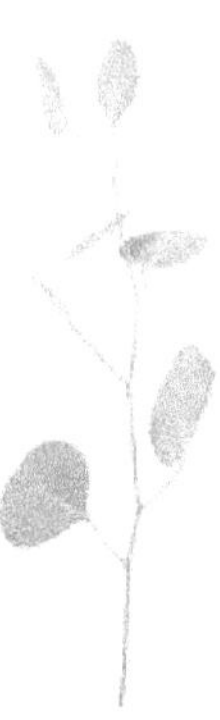

Simply mix one part of lemon eucalyptus oil with ten parts of witch hazel or sunflower oil to create your own natural mosquito repellent. It is notable here that the scientific researchers of the University of Florida caution against using this natural mosquito repellent on children of less than three years or age.

2. **Lavender:**

Another natural mosquito repellent is the scent and oil produced by the crushed lavender flowers. You can even grow lavender in your indoor and outdoor planters. Simply pluck the flowers and crush them to take out the oil. Apply this oil on your skin to prevent mosquitoes from biting you. Otherwise, you can also drop some drops of this oil on a clean, soft cloth and rub it against your skin.

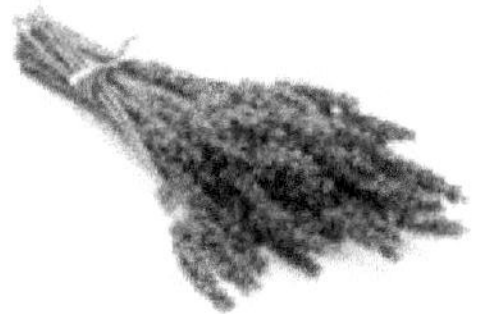

It also contains antiseptic and analgesic qualities as well therefore it soothes and calms your skin along with preventing the mosquitoes from biting it.

3. **Cinnamon Oil:**

Cinnamon oil is considered to be great topper to oatmeal and applesauce. A scientific study carried out in Taiwan proves that it has the ability to kill mosquito eggs. It also repels adult mosquitoes especially the Asian tiger mosquito. It is notable here that a concentrated cinnamon oil can be irritating on your skin so you need to be careful in applying it.

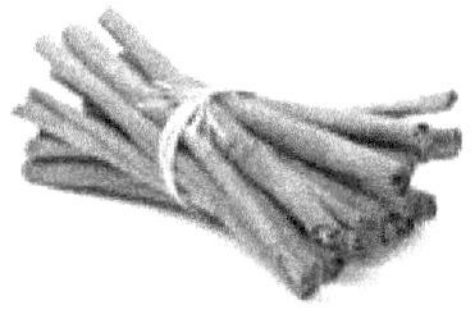

You can make a diluted solution of this natural mosquito repellent by mixing 24 drops of lavender oil per 4 ounces of water. Simply spray this solution on your ski, clothing, plants and around the house.

4. **Thyme Oil:**

Thyme oil is the best natural mosquito repellent present out there in the nature. A scientific study was conducted in which hairless mice were applied with 5% thyme oil and it provided a 95% prevention rate.

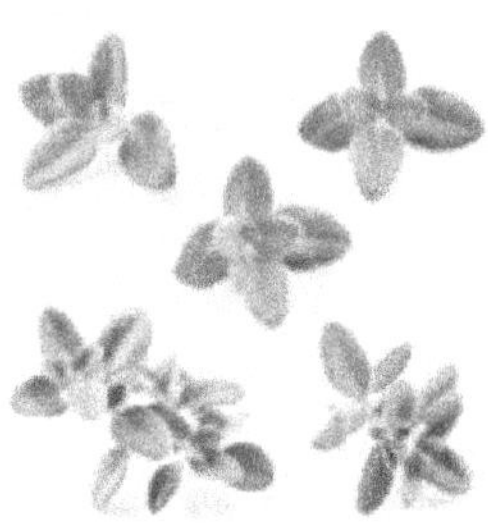

To make a solution, mix 4 drops of thyme oil with a teaspoon of any base oil such as jojoba and olive oil. To make a spray, mix 2 ounces of water with 5 drops of thyme oil.

5. **Greek Catnip Oil:**

It is a part of mint family and it is a great mosquito repellent. It grows an 18 inches long white and pink flowers but the oil is extracted from its leaves.

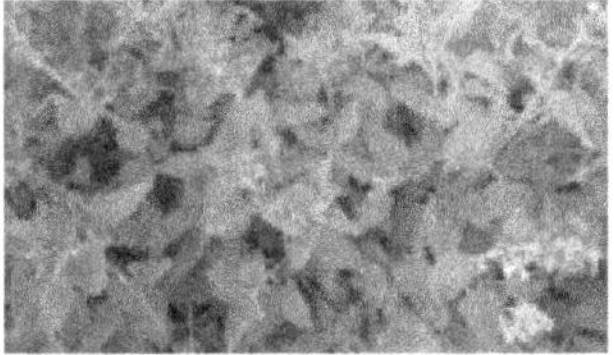

A scientific study has proven that this oil can effectively repel mosquitoes from two to three hours. It is also considered to 10% more effective than any DEET based chemical mosquito repellent.

6. **Soybean Oil:**

Medical Entomology Laboratory at University of Florida has proven through a scientific study that in comparison to citronella based products any soybean based product provides longer lasting prevention from mosquitoes.

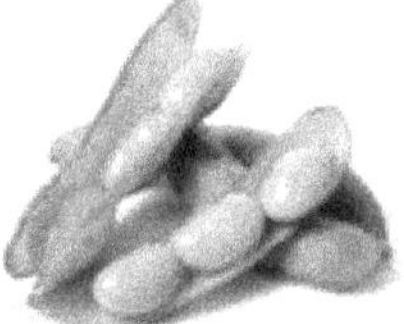

You can also add a bit of lemon grass oil in it to make a home mixture. This combination provides protection against a number of different species of mosquitoes.

Although all of these oils are extracted from different parts of many plants but applying them in higher concentration can harm your skin. Therefore, it is pertinent to make a diluted solution of these oils with water, lotion or any base oil such as olive oil. It is also recommended that you take a spot test on a patch of your skin before deciding to use any of these oil mosquito repellents on your skin. It will tell you about the allergies you can have from these kinds of natural repellents. Do this test two to three days before starting to use any of the above mentioned natural remedies against mosquito bites. If you find any kind of allergies on your skin by its use, you must immediately stop using this oil and wash your skin. You must also go to the local poison control center to get sure that any poison has not been spread in your blood by the usage.

Chapter 3: Homemade Insect Repellents for Pets

Spring season is wet and cold in most of the zones on this planet. This is the time when mosquitoes spread real fast and feed on the blood of other living being around them. This increases the rate of spread of diseases as well. To prevent all this from happening, you must decrease the growth of mosquitoes at the first place and preventing the spread of diseases through them in the second place.

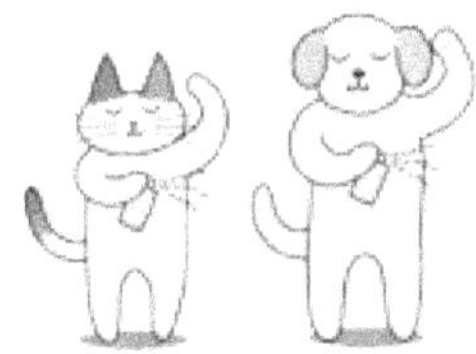

These nuisance bugs are a constant headache for you and your pets. Preventing mosquito bite prevention helps you gain prevention against the spread of heartworm in your pets as well. There are a number of effective ways through which you can protect your pets from the gruesome bites of dangerous mosquitoes.

1. **Lemon Eucalyptus Oil:**

    It is the most effective natural mosquito repellent to protect your pets. It has been registered with the U.S. Environmental Protection Agency along with DEET based chemical repellents and picaridin. This means that the product has been thoroughly examined and completely approved to be used safely by humans and their pets.

The Center of Disease Control and Prevention has also recommended its use to prevent from the mosquitoes that carry West Nile Virus in their bites.

Natural repellents for your pets are prepared the same way. There are certain collars available in the market as well that contain the essential oils to protect your dog and prevent mosquito bites. You can just simply put that collar in your pet's neck and voila! The problem has been solved.

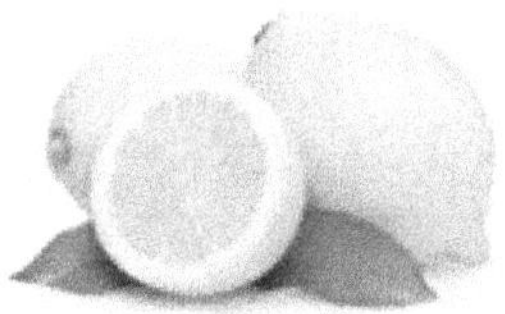

2. **Geranium Oil and Soybean Oil:**

Bite blocker is considered to be a natural mosquito repellent because it contains the geranium and soybean oils. A scientific study conducted by the New England Journal of Medicine Study has proved that it provides upto 94.6 minutes prevention of mosquito bites.

Another scientific study conducted by the United States Department of Agriculture has also ranked the products containing geranium and soybean oils as number two for preventing mosquito bites.

Bite blocker is available in geranium, soybean and coconut oils. It is also available in market in the form of pet sprays.

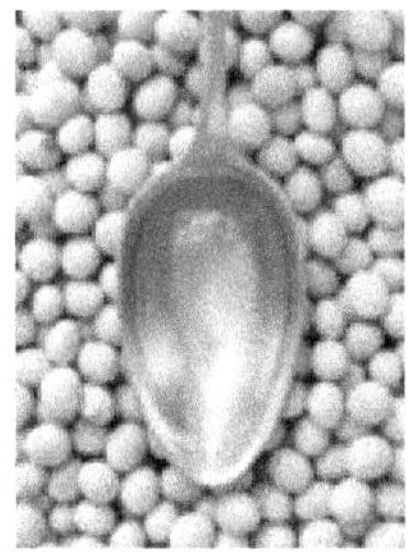

3. **Citronella:**

It is very well known mosquito repellent. Oils are extracted from the plant of Citronella and used to make sprays, lotions and candles with the power of repelling mosquitoes.

A scientific study conducted by the University of Guelph has assessed that the effectiveness of 5% citronella incense and 3% citronella candles in preventing mosquito bites on both human and their pets. It further provided the details that subjects positioned next to citronella incense suffered 24.2% and subjects positioned next to citronella candles suffered 42.3% less mosquito bites.

Therefore, basing on these studies, the citronella candles must not be used as standalone mosquito repellent but in a combination with other topical repellents. It is also available in market in the form of pet sprays.

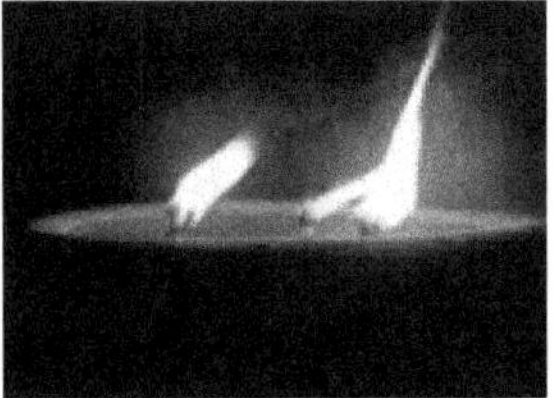

4. **Fennel Oil:**

A scientific study conducted at the Seoul National University in Korea has suggested that any mosquito repellent spray containing 5% fennel oil has proved to be 84% more effective in preventing the bites for upto 90 minutes whereas any repellent body cream with 8% fennel oil is proved to be 70% more effective in protecting the skin of both yourself and your pets from the gruesome bites of mosquitoes. It is also available in market in the form of pet sprays.

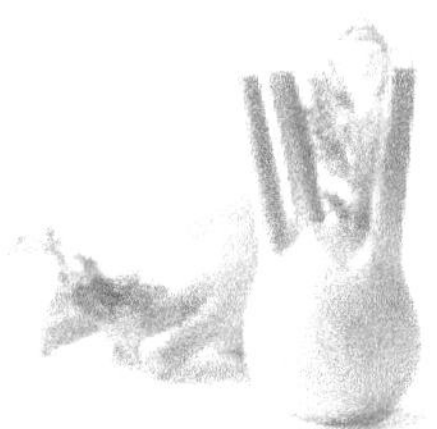

5. **Clove Oil:**

Two scientific studies have proven that undiluted clove oil is highly effective as a mosquito repellent. However, you must not apply undiluted clove oil on your pet's skin without diluting it because it can be harmful to the skin otherwise. It is a great homemade mosquito repellent. It is also available in market in the form of pet sprays.

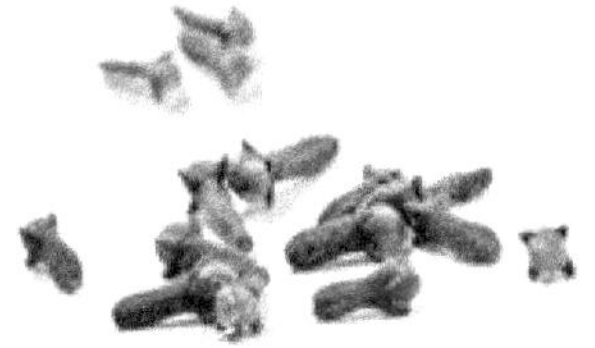

6. **Celery Extract:**

A scientific study conducted at Thailand compared a tropical extract of celery with 15 different kinds of mosquito repellents. The results proved that the celery extract does not burn the skin and cause irritation in it. It is also found to be active against the 25% DEET formula. It is also available in market in the form of pet sprays.

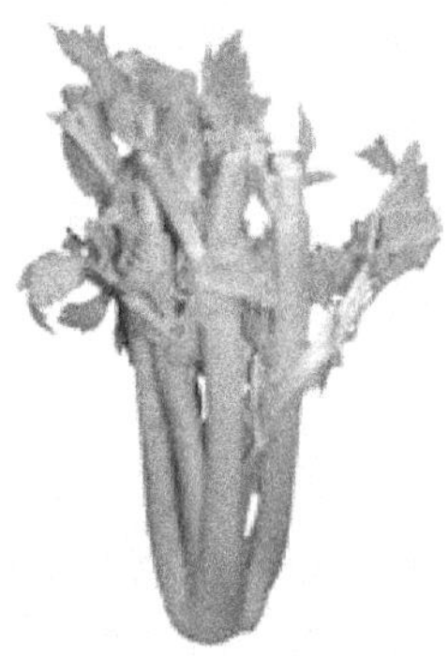

7. **Neem Oil:**

Azadirachtins is an insecticidal compound found in the leaves of a neem tree. It is a great mosquito repellent if used by mixing coconut oil in it. Rubbing pure neem oil on your skin is not going to give a very pleasant sensation in hot and humid climates.

And yes! Neem oil does not have the smell of roses as well. It is also available in market in the form of pet sprays.

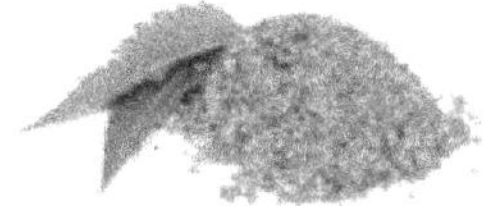

8. **Garlic:**

Garlic is a great vegetable. It has many health benefits. One popular theory suggests that ingesting garlic can provide you and your pet prevention from mosquito bites. A scientific study conducted at the University of Connecticut has examined this theory as double blinded, randomized and placebo controlled cross study.

Therefore, the remedy is not considered to be an effective one as it does not provide a good quantity of prevention against mosquito bites outside the laboratory.

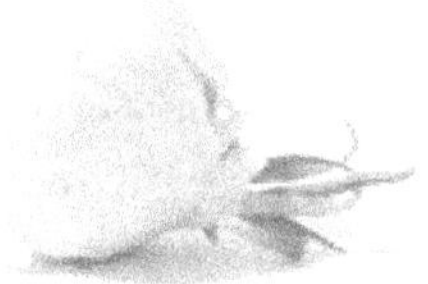

You can use these and many other homemade and natural mosquito repellents to protect both you and your pets from the gruesome bites and the resultant diseases.

Chapter 4: Natural Remedies to Treat Insect Bites

We all just love summer. It brings sunlight, fruity drinks, flirty dresses and insects! All of these insect bites can just kill your mood in no time. Many kinds of bug repellents are used to prevent such bites but they cannot provide around the clock protection anyway. And those clever mosquitoes get the chance to take a bite or more of your (yummy) skin.

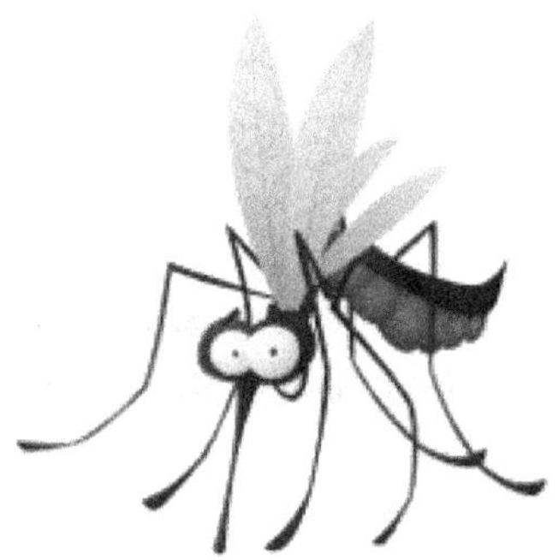

Therefore, the fair chances of getting mosquito bites in summer are quite higher. And if you are the victim this time then just don't lure to the drugstore immediately. There are a number of homemade or natural remedies that you can do to treat these itchy gifts from those summer fellows. These amazing alternatives to chemical treatments and over-the-counter medicines are great in soothing down your pain.

Essential Oils:

There are so many essential oils that work miracles to sooth down the instant pain, itching and swelling after a brutal mosquito bite such as tea tree, coconut and lavender oils. Tea tree oil is particularly an antibacterial as well therefore it provides you a good account of protection from the bacteria being delivered on to your skin through the mosquitoes as well and thus it prevent infections from incessant scratching.

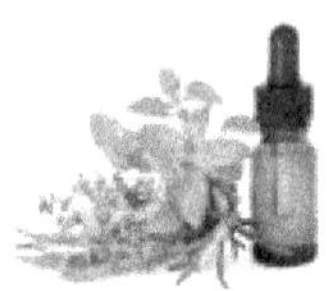

Essential oils are available in the markets under different brands but these can be more acidic than others. Therefore, it is pertinent for you to ask the storekeeper or consult your dermatologist about the concentration of the essential oils before using any on your skin. Strong oil can be diluted with water and thus applied on your skin without any hesitation.

Honey:

Honey, by nature, is anti-inflammatory and thus makes instant itching after a mosquito bite quite less tempting. If you don't mind its stickiness then honey is your new friend for soothing down the instant pain and itching after a mosquito's gruesome attack on your skin.

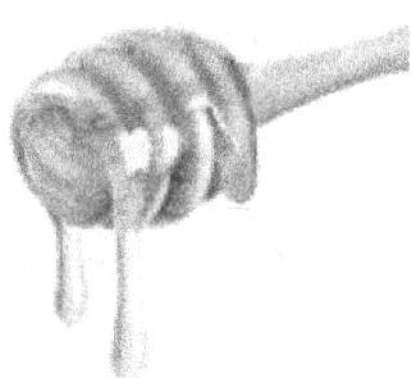

Simply apply honey on the mosquito bite directly after the attack. It will stop the temptation of itching on the area of skin.

Milk and Water:

If you have gone under the unfortunate event of a mosquito bite and don't know what kind of herb or natural oil you must apply on it then simply turn to milk. It is the Mother Nature's first gift to a human being and it keeps on nourishing and soothing them in one way or the other.

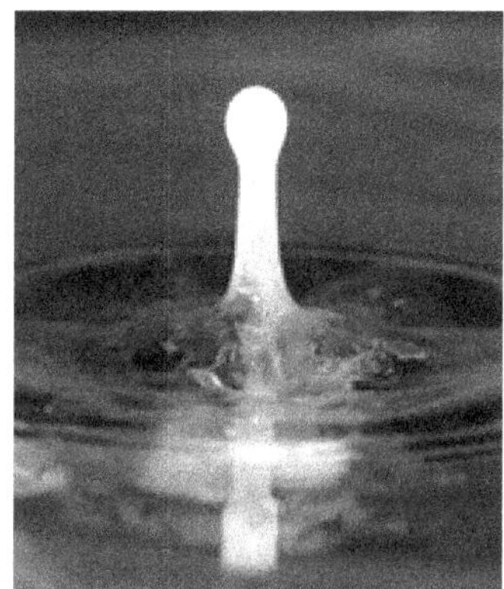

Simply mix equal part of skimmed milk in equal part of water and make a solution. Dip a thin clean cloth in the mixture. A handkerchief or T-shirt works the best. Dab your skin with this concoction. It will sooth your skin immediately.

Lemon or Lime Juice:

Lemon is powerhouse. This fruit contains qualities of an antibacterial agent. Therefore, it provides immediate relief from an itching resultant from the mosquito bite.

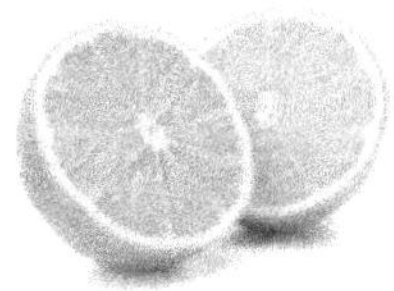

Apply lemon or lime juice on the mosquito bite but it is pertinent to remember that these fruits are acidic and ca burn your skin if applied in direct sunlight therefore stay inside when applying it on your skin.

Toothpaste:

Most of the brands make toothpastes with mint or peppermint flavor. A cooling sensation and feeling of relief is created on your skin by this menthol ingredient.

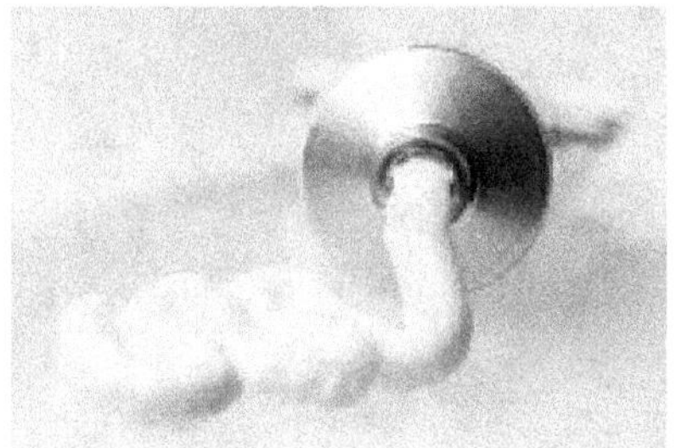

If you apply toothpaste containing mint or peppermint flavor on the mosquito bite then it will give your skin the cooling sensation. And your brain picks up the feeling of cooling sensation more quickly than the itching effect of the mosquito bite. It also helps you reducing the swelling due to its intrinsic astringency.

Basil:

Basil is an amazing kitchen herb. But its uses are not limited to your kitchen only. Basil leaves contain a special chemical that creates a cooling effect on your skin. Camphor is the cooling chemical found in its leaves. It is similar to menthol and peppermint in its effect.

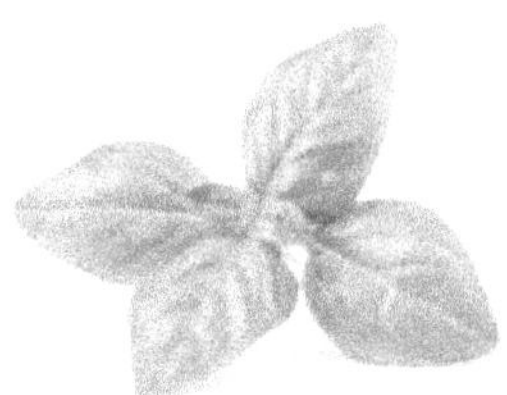

To sooth itching from the mosquito bite instantly, crush a few leaves of basil and apply them directly on the spot.

Ice:

Ice has the power of constricting things. It does the same with your body. It constricts the blood vessels and decreases the histamine release in your body. This quality makes it an amazing pain reliever.

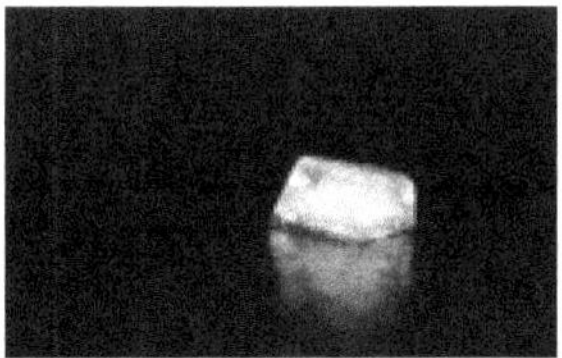

Placing a single ice cube directly on the mosquito bite instantly relieves the pain and sooths down the itching and swelling.

Tea Bags:

Cold tea bags also help you in relieving the pain and itching on your skin from a brutal mosquito bite. They draw out the water and sooths your skin.

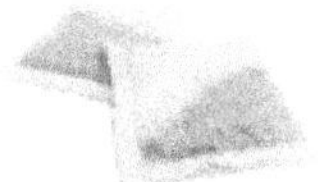

Vinegar:

It is found in every kitchen. And it has unlimited uses. One of them is relieving your skin from the mosquito bites as well. Due to its small acidic levels, it blocks itching on your skin.

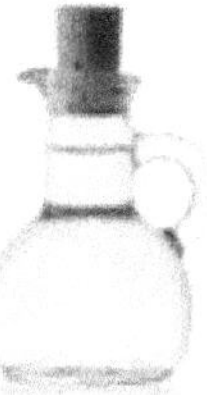

Simply dab a clean thing cloth in vinegar and rub it on the mosquito bite. You can also add three cups of vinegar in warm water tub and take a dip in it if your skin has become the buffet for the mosquitoes last night.

It is the summer time and you need to protect your skin from sunlight. Therefore staying in shady areas is your preference these days but these places are abundant in all types of mosquitoes. They love to feast on your skin. This feasting can gift you itching, pain and swelling all the once. There are a number of homemade remedies and natural ingredients that can help in reliving your skin from the bites. And they are amazing!

Chapter 5: Natural Hacks to Keep Insects Away from Your Home

Despite being tiny and small creatures, mosquitoes can be quite irritating and frustrating even if they don't any means to reach your skin and feast on it. They cause several fatal and dangerous diseases like malaria, yellow fever and dengue in human by landing the germs on your skin.   Several kinds of DEET based chemical mosquito are found in the market. These products are quite good in keeping your soundings mosquito-free however they are quite dangerous to our environment at the same time. Therefore, it is a green thing to adopt natural remedies and homemade recipes to protect yourself and your environment from mosquitoes and the negative effects.

Here we are discussing some of the natural ingredients and homemade recipes in getting rid of mosquitoes in eco-friendly manner. Let's try them!

Dry Ice:

Humans exhale carbon-dioxide and mosquitoes get attracted to it. That is why they find us and then feast on our skin. Dry ice emits carbon-dioxide as well.

Placing dry ice in a container in the room on a little distance from you can attract mosquitoes towards it rather than letting them being drawn to your skin. Keep an eye on the container and as soon as mosquitoes start gathering around the dry ice, you simply shut its lid down. It is a little consuming trick but it is an effective method to drive mosquitoes away from you.

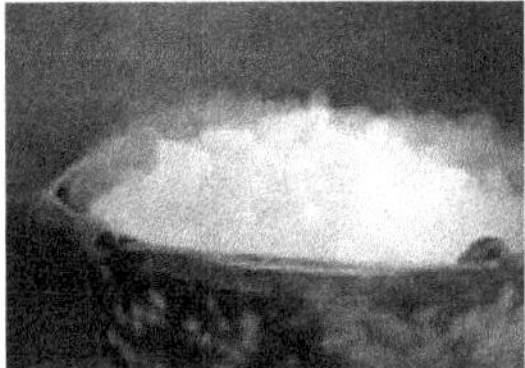

Coffee Grounds:

Stagnant water is a beloved home for mosquitoes to lay their eggs. Therefore, never let water stand in front and inside of your home. This will let no mosquitoes to hoard in your house. However, if somehow you get stagnant water in your surroundings, simply grab a bottle of coffee beans and sprinkle them on it. The coffee beans will force the eggs to come out on the surface of the water and coming on the surface will deprive them of oxygen. Thus they will be killed before hatching and you will become able to prevent mosquito breeding in your house and its surroundings.

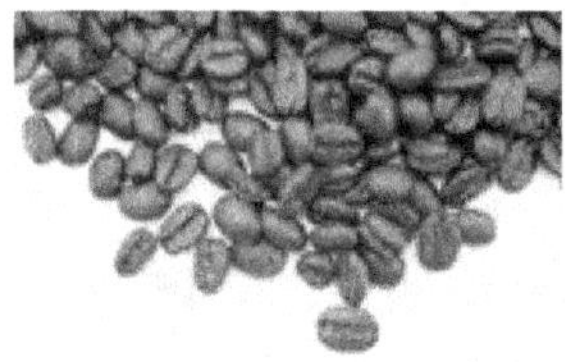

Mosquito Traps:

Mosquito traps are also very effective in killing insects. You can either buy it from the local market or make them at your home. If you want to make it at home then you need an empty plastic bottle. Cut it in half. In a separate bowl, mix brown sugar in warm water and mix the solution well. When properly mixed, pour the mixture into the half cut bottle piece.

It is the time to add yeast in this mixture. Now add the funnel part of the bottle back into it by placing it upside down. Wrap this bottle with a black tape but leave the upper portion of the funnel part uncovered. Now place it in a mosquito prone area. And let it trap all the mosquitoes in it. Change the solution after every fortnight.

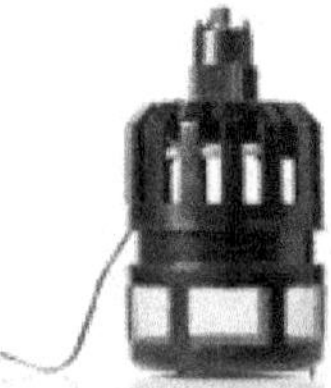

Camphor:

To get rid of the mosquitoes in an environment friendly way is to use camphor. It is a little green tree that you can grow in your home garden as well. Take out some of its leaves and light it in a room after closing all of the doors and windows. Leave it in there for half an hour. Go back in that room and you will find no mosquitoes in there. Enjoy an eco friendly mosquito-free zone!

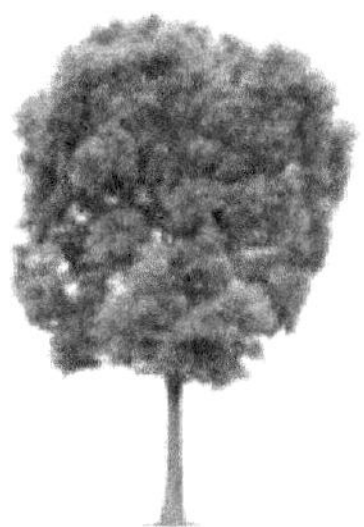

Garlic:

Garlic is a vegetable with a very strong odor. Many humans don't like its smell. Mosquitoes are the same. They also don't abhor its odor. This makes it an effective mosquito repellent for your home.

Simply crush a few pieces of garlic and boil them in hot water. Let it cool down. Then pour it in a spray bottle and sprinkle it all around your home. This will repel all the mosquitoes and your house will become safe.

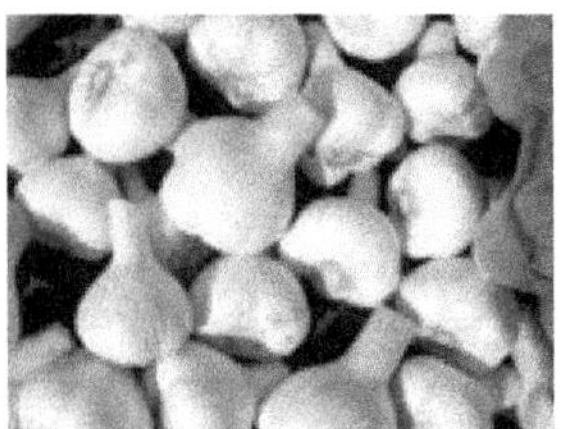

Mint:

Mint is a perennial herb loved by many for its soothingly sweet odor. However, this odor is loathed by mosquitoes. You can either extract its oil from the plant or buy it from the market. Pour the mint oil in a spray bottle and sprinkle it around the house.

Specifically sprinkle in mosquito abundant dark areas of your home. You can also apply it on your skin. You can also grow it in your garden. Its odor will repel the mosquitoes anyway.

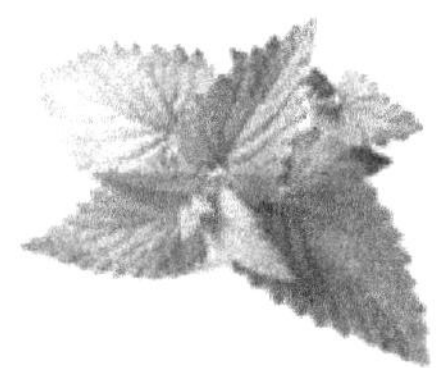

Red Cedar Mulch:

Make red cedar mulch for your garden plants and also use it inside your home to drive away the mosquitoes in an environment friendly manner. This is quite a good remedy and is very easy to adopt as well. Simply take a small bowl of red cedar mulch and boil it in water. On cooling down, pour this solution into a garden sprayer and sprinkle it everywhere in and out of your house. This will hold the mosquitoes away from your eco friendly home.

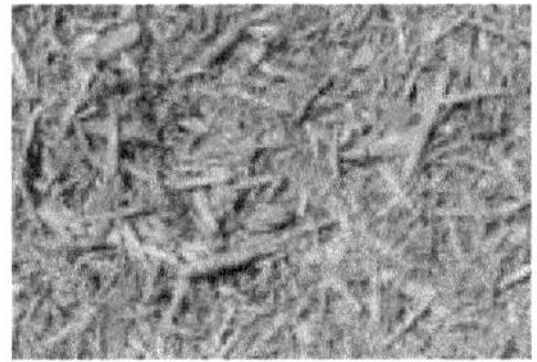

Pinion Wood:

Another environment friendly method to keep mosquitoes away from your house is to gather some pinion wood and burn them outside your home. It will produce a pungent odor. This odor is not adhered by mosquitoes and they get killed. This prevents them from entering in your house.

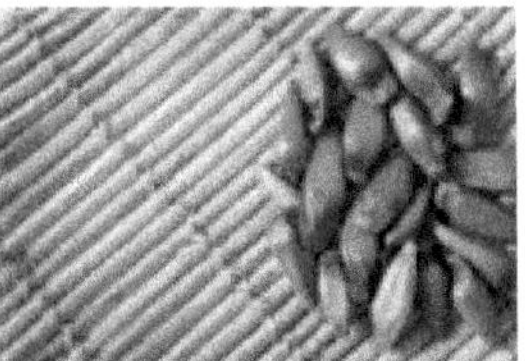

You can use any of these natural remedies to repel mosquitoes away from your house.

Conclusion

Summer is the most beautiful season of the year. It brings a lot of colors, flirty dresses, fancy drinks and insects! All kinds of insects and bugs grow and breed in this season therefore you can find them hanging around in your garden, flying in your house and resting in your bedroom as well. Many effective chemical based repellents are available in markets.

These repellents work greatly in killing these insects and bugs but they have harmful effects on our environment. Therefore, it is highly recommended to adopt organic and natural methods to kill and eliminate these insects from your surroundings.

There are a large number of herbs, ornamental plants and carnivorous plants that you can grow in your garden to repel them. You can also extract oils, crush their leaves and boil them in water to make a number of effective environment friendly mosquito and other insect repellents.

FREE Bonus Reminder

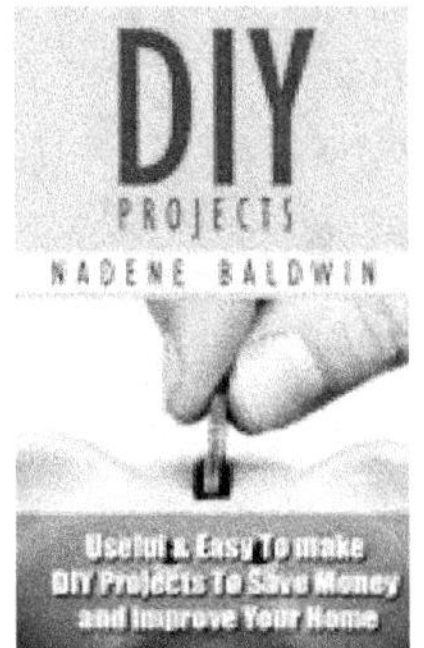

If you have not grabbed it yet, please go ahead and download your special bonus report *"DIY Projects. 13 Useful & Easy To Make DIY Projects To Save Money & Improve Your Home!"*

Simply Click the Button Below

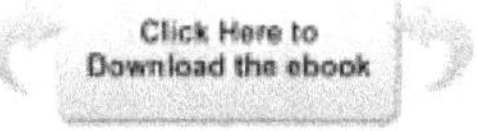

OR **Go to This Page**

http://diyhomecraft.com/free

BONUS #2: More Free & Discounted Books

Do you want to receive more Free & Discounted Books?

We have a mailing list where we send out our new Books when they go free or with a discount on Kindle. Click on the link below to sign up for Free & Discount Book Promotions.

=> Sign Up for Free & Discount Book Promotions <=

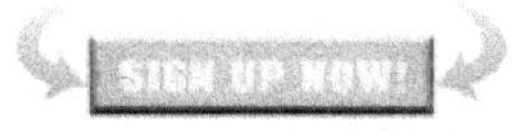

OR Go to this URL

http://zbit.ly/1WBb1Ek